LET THEM GO FREE

A Guide to Withdrawing Life Support

Thomas A. Shannon
&
Charles N. Faso, O.F.M.

GEORGETOWN UNIVERSITY PRESS
Washington, D.C.

As of January 1, 2007, 13-digit ISBN numbers have replaced the
10-digit system.
13-digit Paperback: 978-1-58901-140-3
10-digit Paperback: 1-58901-140-6

Scripture passages are quoted from *The New American Bible*
(New York: P. J. Kennedy & Sons, 1970).

Georgetown University Press, Washington, D.C.

Library of Congress Cataloging-in-Publication Data

Shannon, Thomas A. (Thomas Anthony), 1940–
  Let them go free : a guide to withdrawing life support /
Thomas A. Shannon and Charles N. Faso.
        p.   cm.
  ISBN 1-58901-140-6 (pbk. : alk. paper)
    1. Life-support systems (Critical care)   2. Medical ethics.
  3. Euthanasia.   I. Faso, Charles N.   II. Title. [DNLM: 1. Decision
  Making.   2. Euthanasia, Passive.   3. Catholicism.   4. Family.
  5. Life Support Care.   6. Pastoral Care.   7. Withholding
  Treatment. WB 60 S528L 2007]

  RC86.7S53   2007
  179.7—dc22   2006021490

∞This book is printed on acid-free paper meeting the requirements of
the American National Standard for Permanence in Paper for Printed
Library Materials.

14 13 12 11 10 09 08 07   9 8 7 6 5 4 3 2
First printing

Printed in the United States of America

*This book is dedicated to the
memory of our parents*

*John E. and Clara J. Shannon
and
Joseph C. and Isabel L. Faso*

Contents

v

Introduction

In our world we have decisions, options, and choices that previous generations simply could not imagine. As a result, we may feel that we have no traditions or precedents on which we can rely to resolve these new situations, and so we have to find our own way.

The process of dying is surely one of those situations of our time that presents difficulties for us. In a time when life was harder but less complex, people did not have the choices we have and did not have to do what we often need to do when someone close to us is dying. In earlier days people did not live as long as we do now; to reach thirty or forty years was considered to be a ripe old age. The causes of this were many: lack of sanitation, epidemics that had no cures or effective containment, poor diets, poverty, and a lack of understanding of the causes of many diseases. Traditional healers provided a context of care and support but there were few remedies. It was not until it was discovered that germs cause disease and the development of vaccines to respond to them, together with dramatic improvements in sanitary and dietary habits, that the first inroads against disease were made. Progress against the major destroyers of human life at an early age was finally identified and managed.

Ironically, we are now suffering from our successes. As a result of enjoying healthier and more varied diets, improved sanitation, a vastly raised quality of life, and the daily advances of modern medicine, humans have a longer life span. But with these advances come new diseases that are proving difficult to cure and that cause gradual debilitation of the individual. The fields of medicine and engineering have combined to provide us with tremendous resources to respond to trauma and organ failure, compensate for the body's functions during massive surgery, and assist in recovery and rehabilitation. But frequently these marvelous technologies bring burdens as well as benefits. They can support, they can compensate, they can even replace bodily and organ functions, but they cannot cure a diseased or failed organ or body.

To acknowledge the limits of medicine is not to criticize or reject it. To recognize limits is a sign of wisdom, even though the consequences may be difficult to accept. But we must not ask of technology, medicine, or the team of physicians and nurses to do more than they can. Sometimes therapy is started or a life support system is put into place to solve an immediate problem such as to respond to an emergency, to provide support after a trauma or surgery, or to compensate for the failure of an organ. Such therapies can be immensely helpful but sometimes the body does not respond, the organ systems do not rally, and patients stay where they are. The machines and life support systems compensate for the failed organ or system, but no curing takes place, no recovery occurs, no rehabilitation takes place. Nothing changes.

This is a particular problem of our modern culture. In earlier times, death came rather swiftly; no medicines or technologies held off its awesome power. But now we have technical capacities to hold back death—at least for a time. The capacity to prolong life through the use of technology surely fills us with awe, just as surely as does the power to end that process by withdrawing these technologies. We need to rethink our traditions to guide us in times of anxiety, help us in a new medical context, and comfort us in our sorrow.

As an aid in responding to these new situations, we have written this guide for difficult times of decision making, possibly one of the most difficult and painful decisions anyone has to make in their entire lives: the decision to remove a life support system from a loved one. We offer this guide for two reasons. First, it provides a way for you to think through what you are doing. The questions and discussions offered are a way to examine your options, to clarify what you are doing, and to help you develop a sense of your responsibilities and your limits. Second, we offer a family prayer service that can be used before the life support system is withdrawn. We know that prayers often help a family get through a difficult situation, but more importantly, prayers express our dependence on God and place us within the community of God's people. We should not be alone when we decide to withdraw a life support system. Our hope is that this prayer service will ensure the presence of at least a small community to assist you in making and carrying out your decision.

Many other families have been in your situation. They have had to consider what to do, and frequently they have had to do it alone. These families have followed their instincts, and they have done what they thought best. But perhaps they didn't always know that other families have had to do the same thing. We hope that by sharing the thoughts that people often think about as they struggle with this decision will make you feel less alone during this difficult time.

What Should You Do?

*O*ne of the hardest things to do when families are faced with the possibility of withdrawing a life support system is trying to figure out what to do. You are in a time of stress and anxiety, you have not had to do this before, and you simply may not know what questions to ask. Your sorrow and anxiety are compounded by a feeling of being out of control because you understand that the decision to remove a life support system begins the grieving process over the death of the patient, your loved one. We hope that the following questions and discussions will assist you in your decision making.

What Is the Patient's Medical Condition?

It is important for you to know the person's medical condition because accepting this situation is the basis on which many other decisions will be made. Thus it is critical to make sure that you obtain as much information as you need from the physician and that you receive it in a language you understand. Don't be afraid to ask him or her to repeat something or to explain it in a different way or to ask for an interpreter; the stakes are obviously high.

Sometimes individuals become confused in an intensive care unit. These units are very busy and frequently noisy places. There is a lot of equipment, much of it attached to the patient, and it can be difficult to understand what it all means. Sometimes the equipment can interfere with communicating with your relative, or you may be afraid to touch your relative because you think you might disturb or set off some of the equipment. You may not know how to tell the difference between an alarm that sounds an emergency call and the normal sounds the machines make when monitoring the patient's condition. Be sure to talk over these feelings, fears, and concerns with the staff because although they are used to everything that goes on in the unit you are not. Share your questions and your problems with them; they are there to help the patient and the family.

Also—and this is a difficult and delicate issue— in your roles as family members worried about your relative's medical condition, you may hear what you want to hear or in your minds you may emphasize words you want to hear. However, your hopes and desires must be reconciled with the facts of the situation, and although you never want to despair, you need to accept the limits of medicine and technology and the facts of the patient's condition. Thus, you must try to be honest about the situation, be open to hear what is being said, and form a clear vision that allows you to see reality rather than what you want to see.

To attain this high level of acceptance and control is difficult, and it does not—nor should it—come at once. Everyone needs time to search, to ask, to confront, to deny, to be angry and sad, and finally, to accept. You need time to let the reality and enormity of the situation enter in so you can face it and come to terms with it. The first major step in this process of acceptance and decision making is understanding the medical realities for the patient.

What Are the Medical Options?

Once you have a sense of the medical condition of the patient, you can then begin to examine how to respond to that situation. It is important to remember to be guided by your desire to care for the patient and to show your love for him or her.

Again, the physician can be an important resource at this point. Physicians have a vast range of experience and expertise that can be brought to bear on the particular condition of the patient, and they will help you understand the different possibilities for treatments and outcomes. The physician can also help to sort out the many options that may theoretically be available, although only some of them might actually be appropriate for the patient. It is important to understand what the proposed treatment or technology will actually do. You can ask questions such as, will the proposed treatment or therapy help cure the patient? Will it help restore the patient to where he or she was, healthwise, before this illness? Will the treatment maintain the present condition of the patient? Or does the technology prolong the dying process? These questions are difficult to ask and answers to them are not always easy to accept. But they are important because the answers can help you understand what will benefit the patient and can lead you to determine whether the treatment will help the patient recover or whether the therapy will simply maintain the patient's present condition and not really benefit him or her.

Sometimes it is the case that a therapy or technology will not improve a patient's condition. This is not the fault of the physicians or the technology. It is simply a limit—a limit of the physical body and a limit of medical treatment—that you need to accept. For example, a respirator cannot repair damaged lungs but it can assist the lungs while the patient receives therapy. You also need to keep in mind that while it may seem that there are numerous options, many of these may not be appropriate for the patient. So, along with receiving guidance from the physician, it is important to have a clear understanding of the therapy and its limits. Once you have a good sense of the patient's medical condition and the options that are beneficial, then you can examine other critical questions in determining how best to care for the patient.

Has the Patient Said Anything about His or Her Treatment Wishes?

One way to help people best is to enable them to realize their wishes or desires, and this can also be the case with desperately ill relatives. Before a person enters the hospital, he or she may discuss what they want or don't want for treatment. Sometimes these discussions are casual or informal and are spurred by reading a newspaper story or seeing a television show about someone else. In response the person may say, "I don't want that done to me," or "That's the way I'd like to be cared for." These moments are illuminating because you can learn what a person's important medical wishes are, and when such moments occur, you should participate in them carefully and thoughtfully.

Other discussions can be more formal, such as when a person drafts an advance directive that specifies what he or she would or would not like done in the event of a health crisis. The advance directive might designate an individual to make decisions and may provide instructions on what to do in various conditions, or the individual might be told to use his or her best judgment.

If an advance directive exists or a designated decision maker is identified, the physician should be made aware of this so that he or she properly plans for the care of the patient. It helps everyone involved to feel better if they know that what is being done is what the patient would want you to do, as painful as that may be.

What If the Patient Hasn't Said Anything about What He or She Wants Done?

Sometimes the illness or hospitalization comes quickly and there hasn't been time to discuss with the patient what he or she would want done. In this case, there are some ways to think about how to care for the patient.

First, you can ask, what looks best for the patient? This is the stage where you find out what the medical condition is and what options are available, and then you can make your most informed judgment about what would be best for the patient. You know that your loved one is ill and you want to do what you can to help him or her. Thus you use this information to find the best course of medical action.

Another important question you can ask is, what do we think he or she would have wanted to do? If you know the patient well, even if you never had a direct conversation about this particular circumstance, you might have a clear sense of how he or she might have approached this situation. This question of what the patient would have wanted to do is frequently asked when the therapy seems only to be maintaining the patient in his or her current condition.

The family of Paul Brophy, a firefighter in Boston who suffered a severe stroke in 1983, responded to the crisis first with an extremely intense and aggressive course of medical therapy. They wanted to provide every opportunity for Paul to recover. But after a while it became clear that the therapies and technologies had reached their limits and would only maintain him rather than cure him or restore him to some measure of independent existence. They knew that they had done the best they could for him and that they had provided the appropriate therapies, medications, and technologies, but nothing had worked. It was at that point that the family began to ask what Paul would have wanted in that situation. Mr. Brophy's family had the knowledge that he did not want to be maintained in his present critical condition. Paul Brophy eventually died in 1986.

Or you could ask, as others do, if I were in that situation, what would I want done? This approach isn't perfect because individuals differ and may want different things. But the approach helps us to see the situation from the patient's perspective and to consider the alternatives from his or her point of view. In this scenario you try to understand what is going on, what the expectations are, what the hopes are. In short, you try to put yourself in the patient's shoes to understand what his or her expectations are and, with that in mind, try to determine what to do.

These approaches help us approximate the patient's wishes and desires and, therefore, allow us to provide appropriate care for him or her. Again, in all of these situations, the experience of the health care team, as well as hospital chaplains, can be invaluable to you as you try to think through what to do. They are there to help you.

Do We Have to Do Everything?

One of the main difficulties that caregivers face in these cases is choosing from among all the different technologies and therapies that are available. New treatments and technologies are continually being developed, so the choices can be overwhelming, especially when a decision must be made quickly.

The first step in deciding what to do is to recognize what you are clearly obliged to do: to care for this particular person. Beyond all doubt and debate, and beyond all consideration of technology capability, love and concern impel you to care for the patient. This is especially true when you are united to this person as a spouse, parent, son, daughter, or friend. Begin your decision-making process by *affirming* your desire to care for and love this special individual in your life.

But does caring mean that you have to use everything medically possible? Not necessarily. It may simply be impossible to do everything. The hospital may not have the technology to do what is possible, or the patient may be in such a weakened physical condition that his or her body will not accept a particular treatment.

Additionally, a common moral tradition in medical ethics recognizes that you are under no obligation to use means that are disproportionate to the goals you seek. That is, you have to look at what the treatment or technology does and determine whether it is a benefit or burden to the patient. If you discover that the treatment or technology will cause a great deal of pain or physical discomfort, if it will expose the patient to a high degree of risk of further harm, if it will not improve the patient's condition, or if it puts an overwhelming financial burden on the patient or family, then one can conclude that a treatment or technology is disproportionate or extraordinary and therefore one has no moral obligation to use it. Even if a proposed treatment is routine or standard, the key moral question must focus on the question of whether the benefits it provides outweigh the burdens it imposes. The focus of moral evaluation should be the effects of the treatment, not the treatment itself.

But you may be uncertain about how much weight to give to the cost of therapy, or you may not be sure how to weigh the patient's will to live with respect to the pain of the procedure. Try to evaluate the situation in light of what you currently know and do your best to show your care and love for the patient. For example, let us consider the procedure of kidney dialysis. Sometimes a person will have a serious kidney disease or the kidneys may have failed as a consequence of another disease. The typical response to this is to provide the patient with dialysis as a means of compensating for the loss of his or her own kidneys or their function. This therapy is effective and can compensate well for the body's inability to excrete waste products of metabolism. If kidney failure is the main health issue, then it might be proper to use dialysis, at least until other issues can be sorted out.

Or consider a person suffering from heart failure. Eventually this condition puts a strain on the kidneys, so dialysis may be suggested. One can ask here whether dialysis will help the person's overall condition or whether it will delay this person's death. In this case, the use of dialysis may be disproportionate because its burdens may outweigh the benefits and it may make no contribution to the patient's recovery.

A simple rule of thumb is to look at what the treatment or therapy does for the patient. Does it help the patient recover? Does it help the patient attain a measurable degree of his or her previous capacities? Or do the therapies and technologies keep the patient in his or her current condition, put him or her in a limbo, or inflict a heavy burden of pain and distress?

Can Therapy Be Stopped Once It Has Been Started?

Starting a therapy or technology is standard procedure in an emergency room: Treat first and ask questions later. Frequently we won't know if a technology or therapy will help until it is tried. We all want to show our care by doing what we think is best for the patient, so standing by and doing nothing during a health crisis can be difficult and frustrating. Just knowing that tests are being performed is often consoling because at least you know that something is being done. But a time comes when the therapies and technologies that have been started do not work, or they do not work as well as had been hoped, or they simply prolong the life of the patient but not the quality of life. The question is then raised about whether one should stop a therapy.

Stopping a therapy or technology is difficult. When the health care team initiates treatments and technologies, it creates a commitment to the patient on the part of the staff. A certain momentum begins to build, efforts are made on behalf of the patient, and expectations can become quite high. Once all this has begun, admitting that the treatment plan is not working, not working well, or is simply maintaining the status quo, is quite difficult. No one likes to admit failure, especially in the medical context where failure to cure frequently means that the patient will not recover. This is the time when your understanding about the medical situation and your ability to be honest about the patient's condition are most difficult but most necessary to put into practice.

In this context it is most important to remember that you do not have to continue treatments or technologies that are disproportionate to the goals you wish to achieve. You can authorize the discontinuation of a therapy when it is reasonably clear that it is not working or that the burdens it imposes are disproportionate to any benefits that the patient might gain. Morally speaking, a decision to end a treatment or technology is justifiable when the intervention is not producing expected benefits, when it is not working, when it is maintaining the patient in limbo, or when it is harming the patient. No one is morally bound to do the impossible, the heroic, or the extraordinary. Withdrawal signifies that nothing more can be done medically, that the patient no longer has the capacity to recover or benefit from the procedures, and that new ways must be found to manifest your love for this special person. Withdrawing therapy signifies the beginning of the grieving or mourning process, and this can make the decision more difficult.

The family of Nancy Cruzan comes to mind in this context. When she was brought into the emergency room after she became unconscious in an automobile accident in 1983, all sorts of emergency procedures were performed. She was appropriately placed on a feeding tube and other support systems to maintain her while other tests were performed and therapies attempted. After several years, however, it became apparent to the family that nothing would restore their daughter to her previous healthy condition, so rather than continue to use disproportionate means and pursue what they understood to be futile therapies, the family asked to have the feeding tube withdrawn. Nancy Cruzan died in December 1990.

In 1990, Terri Schiavo was taken to the hospital after her husband found her unconscious. The health care team initiated various therapies and rehabilitation interventions, including experimental brain treatments, but eventually she was diagnosed as being in a persistent vegetative stage. After several years it became apparent to her husband that she would not recover, and he asked that the feeding tube withdrawn. A bitter court battle with Terri's parents followed but eventually, in March 2005, the feeding tube was withdrawn and she died within a few days.

Both families did what was appropriate, what was necessary, and what was loving and caring for their loved one: They did what was medically indicated. Eventually both of the families had to come to terms with the difficult fact that the best that medicine could offer could not bring their daughter or spouse back to them. In the language of their religious traditions, they asked that the life support system be removed and that the women be put in God's hands.

Knowing that you are doing what is right does not make doing that any easier, however. Stopping a treatment is a difficult decision, but if you know you have done what you can, that you have carefully examined the alternatives, and you are convinced the only means available are extraordinary and do not confer a benefit, then you can make the difficult decision to stop medical intervention with a well-informed and good conscience.

Do I Have to Use Artificial Means of Feeding?

This question raised in the Brophy, Cruzan, and Schiavo cases is exceptionally difficult. A feeding tube is the technical capacity that provides a liquid diet through a tube inserted either through the nose or by surgically implanting the tube directly into the stomach. When persons can no longer feed themselves, eat solid foods, or drink orally, they can be fed this way so their nutritional level is maintained at an appropriate level.

Determining whether you should allow this intervention or continue it is a difficult moral question that admits of no easy answers. Physicians, moral theologians and philosophers, church and civic leaders, as well as our entire culture, are divided on this question, and it is increasingly being brought before the courts. To help you begin to think about such a difficult decision, let's review some of the thinking on both sides of the question. Whereas this discussion probably won't make it any easier for you to make a decision, it may help you review the options and provide you with a point of departure for making your decision.

For those who favor the withholding or withdrawal of such a feeding procedure, we suggest that you consider the following. First, feeding is not a form of medical treatment, and so the moral categories of proportionate or disproportionate forms of therapy cannot be considered. Second, if you do not feed someone, you know what will happen. Therefore, removing the means of feeding someone seems to directly aim at that person's death. Third, providing food and water—even though this is done through a tube—is an expression of the most basic form of care one can show for someone else. While you may not be able to cure the individual, surely you can feed him or her. Finally, by not feeding or providing nutrition to someone in this fashion, are you not taking the first step on the road that will lead to the gradual practice of and acceptance of mercy killing? And if you accept that premise, then once you do this, might there be nothing that would stop you from killing other vulnerable individuals in society?

Those who favor using or continuing the use of a feeding tube suggest the following ideas. First, beyond providing nutritional requirements, does this method of feeding contribute to helping the patient recover? That is, is the patient beyond current medical help and is this means of feeding simply keeping the patient in his or her present condition? Second, is this means of feeding a benefit to the patient? If the patient is in a preterminal coma, in a persistent vegetative stage, or physically debilitated, are you showing your care for the patient by maintaining him or her in that present condition? While feeding a patient is surely good, is it a good to be pursued in light of everything else that is happening to him or her, particularly if there are no medical alternatives left? Third, does the fact that a technology to deliver nutrition exists mandate that you use it? Or do you also have to consider the impact and effects of that technology on the patient? Fourth, since there are some physical consequences associated with artificial feeding, will this cause any harm to the patient? Here, the advice of the physician is very significant. Finally, in your efforts to preserve and maintain physical life, are you not in danger of making physical life your highest value and thereby possibly forgetting that there is a life that transcends the physical and that is more important than our bodily life?

These questions are exceptionally difficult to sort out. Some people may argue that withholding or withdrawing forms of artificial feeding is "playing God," and that by doing this one is exercising a life-and-death power over a patient. On the other hand, it is important not to let technology become our God by conferring on it the power of life and death. You need to exercise your love and care for your loved one in the context of your responsibilities, which are defined by your openness to God, who is the giver of life, and the possibilities and limits that are present in our human capacities.

Considering the decision of whether to provide artificial feeding requires a lot of careful thinking, consultation with the health care team, and a thorough review of the medical status of the patient. It is one thing to consider artificial feeding as part of an overall plan that has reasonable hope of restoring the patient to a healthy condition, but it is quite another thing to understand that the feeding process will simply allow the body to survive, with no benefits, other than the temporary preservation of physical life. If you can make this decision in the context of your love for the patient, a thorough consultation with a variety of people, and your desire to benefit the patient, then the decision will be one that, in the end, you can more easily accept.

What Do I Do if There Are Disagreements?

In even the most ordinary and routine matters of life, one seldom finds total agreement or reasonable consensus. In matters of ultimate concern, you should not be surprised to find disagreement. When considering decisions of this magnitude, make sure that all persons involved have an opportunity to say what they think and that they are listened to. After everyone has had his or her say, the family can determine what common feelings and ideas they share. This is important to do because recognizing areas of common agreement will be important for all future activities. Then the family should state any differences that have been expressed. Do not simply list disagreements, but focus on genuine expressions of feelings of concern. Also, family members should be encouraged to say why they disagree or why they feel the way they do. Awareness and understanding of such concerns may help clarify some of the issues and may make later decisions some-what easier.

Although these discussions will not be easy, they can help develop an atmosphere of cooperation and trust among the family members. Openness and trust among the caregivers must be made priorities from day one; otherwise, the patient will only be harmed by familial bickering and distrust.

After everything has been discussed—hopefully in an atmosphere of love and trust—eventually a decision must be made. Often there is a designated decision maker, whether by virtue of an advance directive, by being the next of kin, or perhaps by being the oldest sibling. This person typically will engage with family members in discussions, take their feelings into account, and rely on their support. Ultimately, however, this person will be the one to make the decision, and convey it to the physician. In arriving at a decision, though, the decision maker also needs to review the options and consider the interests of the patient. Family members may discover that they agree on the main issues and that, on the basis of this agreement, they can proceed to work with the designated decision maker.

It is critically important as soon as possible for the physician to know who the decision maker is so that he or she will know to whom to turn to in case of emergencies. This is not intended to cut out family members from decision making but to avoid harming the patient by having the physician or staff receive conflicting and contradictory advice. Everyone knows that this is a difficult time for all, so one way to serve the well-being of the patient is for family members to respect the decisions at which they have arrived and that are being conveyed by the designated decision maker. A significant way to demonstrate one's love for the patient is to resolve this issue clearly and quickly. Critical decisions cannot be forced, but maintaining openness and trust among family members at this difficult juncture will benefit each member of the family and will promote the good of the patient.

Sometimes however, a decision cannot be reached and family members may genuinely disagree over what is best. Some in the family may feel that, because of closer involvement with the patient, they know what is best, or some family members may not be able to get to the hospital and may wish to delay decisions until they can arrive. Others may reject the status of the designated decision maker. And sometimes the family may simply be overwhelmed and not know what to do.

Most hospitals have support services in the roles of a social worker, a nurse coordinator, a chaplain, or someone from the psychiatry department. Perhaps a member of the clergy who is close to the family can also help. Sometimes the family has a physician friend who has provided much more than health care to them over the years. In the case where a family needs help in resolving difficult decisions, these individuals could be used as mediators. Or a family may wish to let the attending physician make the decisions either because they genuinely trust him or her, or because they simply don't know what else to do. All of these are ways of resolving the issues of who decides, and families should feel able to choose whatever process they are comfortable with.

What Should I Do about Donating Organs?

The best answer to this question is that you should do whatever you are comfortable doing, in discussion with your loved one or family. If you haven't thought about organ donation, let us offer some perspectives.

There is a real need for organ donation. Many individuals could live normal and long lives if they could receive an organ. There have never been enough organs to help those in need. The major reason why so few people donate organs is that they are seldom asked to do so. We don't usually think about donating organs, so we do nothing about it. And when people are in the situation you find yourselves in now, many doctors and nurses don't like to ask because they know you are under a lot of strain and tension and they don't want to add more difficulties to the situation.

But consider that the gift of an organ can become a source of consolation to a family at a time of sorrow. Many people have found it comforting to know that another life has been preserved or that another family has received a priceless gift. They know and remember that even in death, their loved one was the source of life and health for someone else. Such selfless giving truly expresses the religious ideal of love for neighbor in a very concrete and meaningful way.

If you decide to donate an organ or the organs of your relative, you should know that there will be no disfigurement that will interfere with your plans for a wake. Obviously, a surgical procedure will be necessary to remove the organs, but this will not prevent you from having the memorial service you want. Also, you may be asked to wait a little longer before the ventilator or respirator or other support systems will be disconnected, in order to provide the time to find the recipient and prepare him or her to receive the organs. Depending on when you are able to make this decision, such a delay may be only for a few hours or it may be a day. Reach out to the hospital staff with any and all questions about organ donation. The staff in the hospital will not do anything unless you give your permission.

Conclusion

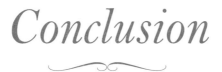

eciding on the medical care for a relative is truly one of the most difficult decisions you will ever have to make. Most of us have to make such decisions with very little preparation or planning. The context of such decision making is filled with tension, fear, guilt, and sadness. Yet we all know that such decisions have to be made, and we all want to do what is best for our relatives and family members.

If you make your decisions in a spirit of love and care for your relatives and if you make them with the understanding that you are trying to do what is best for them and in the recognition of your own limits, you will have done your best for your relatives and you will be loving them as best as you can. Perhaps your decision will be to end a particular treatment or to withdraw a life support system. This is a heartbreaking decision, and after it is made you may feel very alone and sad. We have written a prayer service to help you at this time. We did this because we feel that rituals and prayers are important and because we feel that at this time in particular, few people know exactly what to do or how to act. We hope this prayer service will help you be at peace with your decision, that it will help you in your last moments with your loved one, and that it will provide you with the solace of the grace of God at this time.

The Family
Prayer Service

This prayer service is designed to accompany the withdrawal of a therapy or a life support system. The intent is to provide the support of ritual and prayer and to give some degree of completion and closure for an extremely difficult action. By conducting this service at the bedside with the family, all can affirm their care and concern for their loved one but can also recognize and begin to accept the reality of the limits of human curing and our life here on earth. By joining in prayer at this difficult moment, the family can begin its grieving process and affirm its belief in the living God. By standing in the community of prayer, family members and loved ones can affirm their decision to cease therapy and to release their relative from the bonds that hold her or him from their eternal destiny.

We provide this prayer service as a guide. It is not necessary that all of it be used. The readings and prayers should be adapted to the family and their needs. A family, for example, may wish to offer their own prayers or to select a favorite Bible reading. We propose this prayer service as a format through which a family's needs may be addressed.

MINISTER: Let us join in prayer and open our hearts to the presence of God, the author of life. Let us take comfort in the promise that God is present with those who gather in faith. And let us now pray in the name of the Father, and of the Son, and of the Holy Spirit.

FAMILY: Come, Lord God. Be our strength in this hour, for whether we live or die, we are yours, merciful God, forever.

MINISTER: Lord God, you are the Creator of all life. You allow us the joy of sharing our lives with each other and experiencing your love through our families and friends. We ask you to be with us now and comfort us. We have been blessed with the company and joy of [N.] (insert name) and we take comfort in the memory of those moments. We know you have promised us a greater joy, richer and more lasting than the joy we experience in this life. We wish to gather here as [N.] enters into that joy. We wish to accompany him/her at the beginning of that journey to the place where all tears will be wiped away and sorrow turned to joy.

FAMILY: Amen. We believe in you and your word, O Lord. May you bring [N.] to the joy of your presence.

MINISTER: Let us now listen to the Word of God.

Readings from the Jewish Scriptures

The readings are found on pages 45–50.

Ezekiel 37:1-14. *I shall put my spirit in you, and you shall live.*

Wisdom 3:1-6, 9. *The souls of the virtuous are in the hands of God.*

Wisdom 4:7-15. *A blameless life is a ripe old age.*

Isaiah 25:6–9. *The Lord God will destroy death forever.*

FAMILY: Thanks be to God.

MINISTER: Let us respond to God's Word by praying together Psalm 23.

[1] The LORD is my shepherd; I shall not want.
    [2] In verdant pastures he gives me repose;
Beside restful waters he leads me;
    [3] he refreshes my soul.
He guides me in right paths
    for his name's sake.
[4] Even though I walk in the dark valley
    I fear no evil; for you are at my side
With your rod and your staff
    that give me courage.

[5] You spread the table before me
    in the sight of my foes;
You anoint my head with oil;
    my cup overflows.
[6] Only goodness and kindness follow me
    all the days of my life;
And I shall dwell in the house of the LORD
    for years to come.

Readings from the Christian Scriptures
from the Letters of the Apostles

The readings are found on pages 51–55.

Romans 8:14–23. *We groan while we await the redemption of our bodies.*

1 Corinthians 15:51–57. *Death is swallowed up in victory.*

2 Corinthians 4:14–5:1. *He who raised up the Lord Jesus will raise us up.*

Revelation 21:1–5a, 6b–7. *And there shall be no more death or mourning.*

Minister: This is the Word of the Lord.

Family: Thanks be to God.

Readings from the Gospels

The readings are found on pages 56–61.

> John 11:32-45. *Lazarus, come out.*
>
> Matthew 11:25–30. *Come to me . . . and I will give you rest.*
>
> Luke 23:33, 39–43. *Today you will be with me in paradise.*
>
> John 12:23–26. *If a grain of wheat falls on the ground and dies . . .*
>
> John 14:1–6. *There are many rooms in my Father's house.*

MINISTER: This is the Gospel of our Lord Jesus Christ.

FAMILY: Praise to you, Lord Jesus Christ.

(Silent reflection may follow each scripture reading. A homily may be given after the reading of the Gospel.)

MINISTER: Let us now join in prayer. Word of God, we affirm that you are the beginning and end of all life.

FAMILY: Risen Lord, help us to trust in your promise of life everlasting.

MINISTER: Lord God, you have promised that our lives will be changed and transformed.

FAMILY: Gentle Shepherd, death is hard to accept, but help us to understand that life's journey leads to you.

MINISTER: Source of all goodness, we give you thanks for the blessings which you bestowed on [N.] in this life.

FAMILY: Gracious God, help us to recall the joy and warmth of our times together as we prepare to unbind [N.] and let him/her go free.

MINISTER: Lord Jesus, we recall your command to love and care for one another.

FAMILY: Crucified Lord, help us to understand that while we love, our love has limits and we cannot do everything we want.

MINISTER: God of all creation, strengthen us as we release [N.] from the bonds that hold him/her from you.

FAMILY: Merciful Lord, help us to accept this parting and hold us in your love until we meet again.

MINISTER: Now, Master, you can let your servant go in peace, just as you have promised; because my eyes have seen the salvation which you have prepared for all the nations to see, a light to enlighten the pagans and the glory of your people Israel.

Let us now unbind [N.] and let him/her go free so that he/she may enter into the life that has been prepared for us through the resurrection of Jesus Christ.

FAMILY: Amen. We believe in your Word and the eternal life you have promised to us. We pray that [N.] may now enter this life, free of the bonds that hold him/her from you, our gracious God who awaits him/her with welcoming arms.

The family may now wish to give a final gesture of love or affection for the individual, for example, a kiss, an embrace, or a sign of the cross on the person's forehead. The life support system may be disconnected at this time in the presence of the family while the following prayer is recited. Or the following prayers may be recited by all and then the life support system may be disconnected after the family departs.

Prayer of Commendation

(to be prayed as the life support system is disconnected)

MINISTER: I commend you, my dear brother/sister, to almighty God, and entrust you to your Creator. May you return to him.

FAMILY: Amen.

MINISTER: God of all consolation,
in your unending love and mercy for us
you turn the darkness of death
into the dawn of new life.
Show compassion to your people in their sorrow.
Be our refuge and our strength
to lift us from the darkness of this grief to the peace
and light of your presence.
Your Son, our Lord Jesus Christ, by dying for us,
conquered death, and by rising again, restored
life.
May we then go forward eagerly to meet him, and
after our life on earth
be reunited with our brothers and sisters where
every tear will be wiped away.
We ask this through Christ our Lord.

FAMILY: Amen.

Final Blessing

MINISTER: Blessed are those who have died in the Lord: Let them rest from their labors, for their good deeds go with them. Eternal rest grant unto him/her, O Lord.

FAMILY: And let perpetual light shine upon him/her.

MINISTER: May he/she rest in peace.

FAMILY: Amen.

MINISTER: May his/her soul and the souls of all the faithful departed, through the mercy of God, rest in peace.

FAMILY: Amen.

MINISTER: May the love of God and the peace of the Lord Jesus Christ bless and console us and gently wipe every tear from our eyes: in the name of the Father, and of the Son, and of the Holy Spirit.

FAMILY: Amen.

Readings

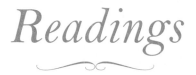

Ezekiel 37:1–14

A reading from the book of the prophet Ezekiel:

¹ The hand of the LORD came upon me, and he led me out in the spirit of the LORD and set me in the center of the plain, which was now filled with bones. ² He made me walk among them in every direction so that I saw how many they were on the surface of the plain. How dry they were! ³ He asked me: Son of man, can these bones come to life? "Lord God," I answered, "you alone know that." ⁴ Then he said to me: Prophesy over these bones, and say to them: Dry bones, hear the word of the LORD! ⁵ Thus says the Lord GOD to these bones: See! I will bring spirit into you, that you may come to life. ⁶ I will put sinews upon you, make flesh grow over you, cover you with skin, and put spirit in you so that

you may come to life and know that I am the LORD. [7] I prophesied as I had been told, and even as I was prophesying I heard a noise; it was a rattling as the bones came together, bone joining bone. [8] I saw the sinews and the flesh come upon them, and the skin cover them, but there was no spirit in them. [9] Then he said to me: Prophesy to the spirit, prophesy, son of man, and say to the spirit: Thus says the Lord GOD: From the four winds come, O spirit, and breathe into these slain that they may come to life. [10] I prophesied as he told me, and the spirit came into them; they came alive and stood upright, a vast army. [11] Then he said to me: Son of man, these bones are the whole house of Israel. They have been saying, "Our bones are dried up, our hope is lost, and we are cut off." [12] Therefore, prophesy and say to them: Thus says the Lord GOD: O my people, I will open your graves and have you rise from them, and bring you back to the land of Israel. [13] Then you shall know that I am the LORD, when I open your graves and have you rise from them, [14] O my people! I will put my spirit in you that you may live, and I will settle you upon your land; thus you shall know that I am the LORD. I have promised, and I will do it, says the LORD.

This is the Word of the Lord. Thanks be to God.

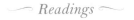

Wisdom 3:1–6, 9

A reading from the book of Wisdom:

[1] But the souls of the just are in the hand of God,
    and no torment shall touch them.
[2] They seemed, in the view of the foolish, to be dead;
    and their passing away was thought an affliction
        [3] and their going forth from us, utter destruction.
But they are in peace.
[4] For if before men, indeed, they be punished,
    yet is their hope full of immortality;
[5] Chastised a little, they shall be greatly blessed,
    because God tried them
    and found them worthy of himself.
[6] As gold in the furnace, he proved them,
    and as sacrificial offerings he took them to
        himself.

[9] Those who trust in him shall understand truth,
    and the faithful shall abide with him in love:
Because grace and mercy are with his holy ones,
    and his care is with his elect.

This is the Word of the Lord. Thanks be to God.

Wisdom 4:7–15

A reading from the book of Wisdom:

[7] But the just man, though he die early, shall be
    at rest.
[8] For the age that is honorable comes not with the
    passing of time,
    nor can it be measured in terms of years.
[9] Rather, understanding is the hoary crown
    for men,
    and an unsullied life, the attainment of
       old age.
[10] He who pleased God was loved;
    he who lived among sinners was transported—
[11] Snatched away, lest wickedness pervert his mind
    or deceit beguile his soul;
[12] For the witchery of paltry things obscures what
    is right
    and the whirl of desire transforms the innocent
       mind.
[13] Having become perfect in a short while, he reached
    the fullness of a long career;
[14]   for his soul was pleasing to the Lord,

therefore he sped him out of the midst of
wickedness.

[15] But the people saw and did not understand,
nor did they take this into account.

This is the Word of the Lord. Thanks be to God.

Isaiah 25:6–9

A reading from the book of the prophet Isaiah:

[6] On this mountain the LORD of hosts will provide for
all peoples

A feast of rich food and choice wines, juicy, rich food
and pure, choice wines.

[7] On this mountain he will destroy the veil that veils
all peoples,

The web that is woven over all nations;

[8] he will destroy death forever.

The Lord GOD will wipe away the tears from all faces;

The reproach of his people he will remove
from the whole earth; for the LORD has spoken.

[9] On that day it will be said:

"Behold our God, to whom we looked to save us!
This is the LORD for whom we looked;
let us rejoice and be glad that he has saved us!"

This is the Word of the Lord. Thanks be to God.

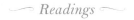

Romans 8:14–23

A reading from the letter of Paul to the Romans:

[14] All who are led by the Spirit of God are sons of God. [15] You did not receive a spirit of slavery leading you back into fear, but a spirit of adoption through which we cry out, "Abba!" (that is, "Father"). [16] The Spirit himself gives witness with our spirit that we are children of God. [17] But if we are children, we are heirs as well: heirs of God, heirs with Christ, if only we suffer with him so as to be glorified with him.

[18] I consider the sufferings of the present to be as nothing compared with the glory to be revealed in us. [19] Indeed, the whole created world eagerly awaits the revelation of the sons of God. [20] Creation was made subject to futility, not of its own accord but by him who once subjected it; yet not without hope, [21] because the world itself will be freed from its slavery to corruption and share in the glorious freedom of the children of God. [22] Yes, we know that all creation

groans and is in agony until now. [23] Not only that, but we ourselves, although we have the Spirit as first fruits, groan inwardly while we await the redemption of our bodies.

This is the Word of the Lord. Thanks be to God.

1 Corinthians 15:51–57

A reading from the first letter of Paul to the Corinthians:

[51] Now I am going to tell you a mystery. Not all of us shall fall asleep, but all of us are to be changed— [52] in an instant, in the twinkling of an eye, at the sound of the last trumpet. The trumpet will sound and the dead will be raised incorruptible, and we shall be changed. [53] This corruptible body must be clothed with incorruptibility, this mortal body with immortality. [54] When the corruptible frame takes on incorruptibility and the mortal immortality, then will the saying of Scripture be fulfilled: "Death is swallowed up in victory." [55] "O death, where is your victory? O death, where is your sting?" [56] The sting of death is sin, and sin gets its power from the law. [57] But thanks be to God who has given us the victory through our Lord Jesus Christ.

This is the Word of the Lord. Thanks be to God.

2 Corinthians 4:14–5:1

A reading from the second letter of Paul to the Corinthians:

[14] [H]e who raised up the Lord Jesus will raise us up along with Jesus and place both us and you in his presence. [15] Indeed, everything is ordered to your benefit, so that the grace bestowed in abundance may bring greater glory to God because they who give thanks are many.

[16] We do not lose heart, because our inner being is renewed each day even though our body is being destroyed at the same time. [17] The present burden of our trial is light enough, and earns for us an eternal weight of glory beyond all comparison. [18] We do not fix our gaze on what is seen but on what is unseen. What is seen is transitory; what is unseen lasts forever.

[1] Indeed, we know that when the earthly tent in which we dwell is destroyed we have a dwelling provided for us by God, a dwelling in the heavens, not made by hands but to last forever.

This is the Word of the Lord. Thanks be to God.

Revelation 21:1–5a, 6b–7

A reading from the book of Revelation:

[1] Then I saw new heavens and a new earth. The former heavens and the former earth had passed away, and the sea was no longer. [2] I also saw a new Jerusalem, the holy city, coming down out of heaven from God, beautiful as a bride prepared to meet her husband. [3] I heard a loud voice from the throne cry out: "This is God's dwelling among men. He shall dwell with them and they shall be his people and he shall be their God who is always with them. [4] He shall wipe every tear from their eyes, and there shall be no more death or mourning, crying out or pain, for the former world has passed away."

[5] The One who sat on the throne said to me, "See, I make all things new!"

[6] "I am the Alpha and the Omega, the Beginning and the End. To anyone who thirsts I will give to drink without cost from the spring of lifegiving water. [7] He who wins the victory shall inherit these gifts; I will be his God and he shall be my son."

This is the Word of the Lord. Thanks be to God.

John 11:32–45

A reading from the Holy Gospel according to John:

[32] When Mary came to the place where Jesus was, seeing him, she fell at his feet and said to him, "Lord, if you had been here my brother would never have died." [33] When Jesus saw her weeping, and the Jews who had accompanied her also weeping, he was troubled in spirit, moved by the deepest emotions. [34] "Where have you laid him?" he asked. "Lord, come and see," they said. [35] Jesus began to weep, [36] which caused the Jews to remark, "See how much he loved him!" [37] But some said, "He opened the eyes of that blind man. Why could he not have done something to stop this man from dying?" [38] Once again troubled in spirit, Jesus approached the tomb.

It was a cave with a stone laid across it. [39] "Take away the stone," Jesus directed. Martha, the dead man's sister, said to him, "Lord, it has been four days now; surely there will be a stench!" [40] Jesus replied, "Did I not assure you that if you believed you would see the glory of God displayed?" [41] They then took away the stone and Jesus looked upward and said:

"Father, I thank you for having heard me.
[42] I know that you always hear me
but I have said this for the sake of the crowd,
that they may believe that you sent me."

[43] Having said this, he called loudly, "Lazarus, come out!" [44] The dead man came out, bound hand and food with linen strips, his face wrapped in a cloth. "Untie him," Jesus told them, "and let him go free."

[45] This caused many of the Jews who had come to visit Mary, and had seen what Jesus did, to put their faith in him.

This is the Gospel of the Lord. Praise to you, Lord Jesus Christ.

Matthew 11:25–30

A reading from the Holy Gospel according to Matthew:

[25] On one occasion Jesus spoke thus: "Father, Lord of heaven and earth, to you I offer praise; for what you have hidden from the learned and the clever you have revealed to the merest children. [26] Father, it is true. You have graciously willed it so. [27] Everything has been given over to me by my Father. No one knows the Son but the Father, and no one knows the Father but the Son—and anyone to whom the Son wishes to reveal him.

[28] "Come to me, all you who are weary and find life burdensome, and I will refresh you. [29] Take my yoke upon your shoulders and learn from me, for I am gentle and humble of heart. Your souls will find rest, [30] for my yoke is easy and my burden light."

This is the Gospel of the Lord. Praise to you, Lord Jesus Christ.

Luke 23:33, 39–43

A reading from the Holy Gospel according to Luke:

³³ When they came to Skull Place, as it was called, they crucified him there and the criminals as well, one on his right and the other on his left.

³⁹ One of the criminals hanging in crucifixion blasphemed him: "Aren't you the Messiah? Then save yourself and us." ⁴⁰ But the other one rebuked him: "Have you no fear of God, seeing you are under the same sentence? ⁴¹ We deserve it, after all. We are only paying the price for what we've done, but this man has done nothing wrong." ⁴² He then said, "Jesus, remember me when you enter upon your reign." ⁴³ And Jesus replied, "I assure you: this day you will be with me in paradise."

This is the Gospel of the Lord. Praise to you, Lord Jesus Christ.

John 12:23–26

A reading from the Holy Gospel according to John:

²³ Jesus answered them:
"The hour has come
for the Son of Man to be glorified.
²⁴ I solemnly assure you,
unless the grain of wheat falls to the earth and dies,
it remains just a grain of wheat.
But if it dies,
it produces much fruit.
²⁵ The man who loves his life
loses it,
while the man who hates his life in this world
preserves it to life eternal.
²⁶ If anyone would serve me,
let him follow me;
where I am,
there will my servant be.
If anyone serves me,
him the Father will honor.

This is the Gospel of the Lord. Praise to you, Lord Jesus Christ.

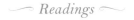
John 14:1–6

A reading from the Holy Gospel according to John:

1 "Do not let your hearts be troubled.
Have faith in God
and faith in me.
2 In my Father's house there are many dwelling places;
otherwise, how could I have told you
that I was going to prepare a place for you?
3 I am indeed going to prepare a place for you,
and then I shall come back to take you with me,
that where I am you also may be.
4 You know the way that leads where I go."
5 "Lord," said Thomas, "we do not know where you
        are going. How can we know the way?"
6 Jesus told him: "I am the way, and the truth, and
        the life;
no one comes to the Father but through me."

This is the Gospel of the Lord. Praise to you, Lord
Jesus Christ.